I0100836

*My name is*

My photograph goes here.

*This is my book.*

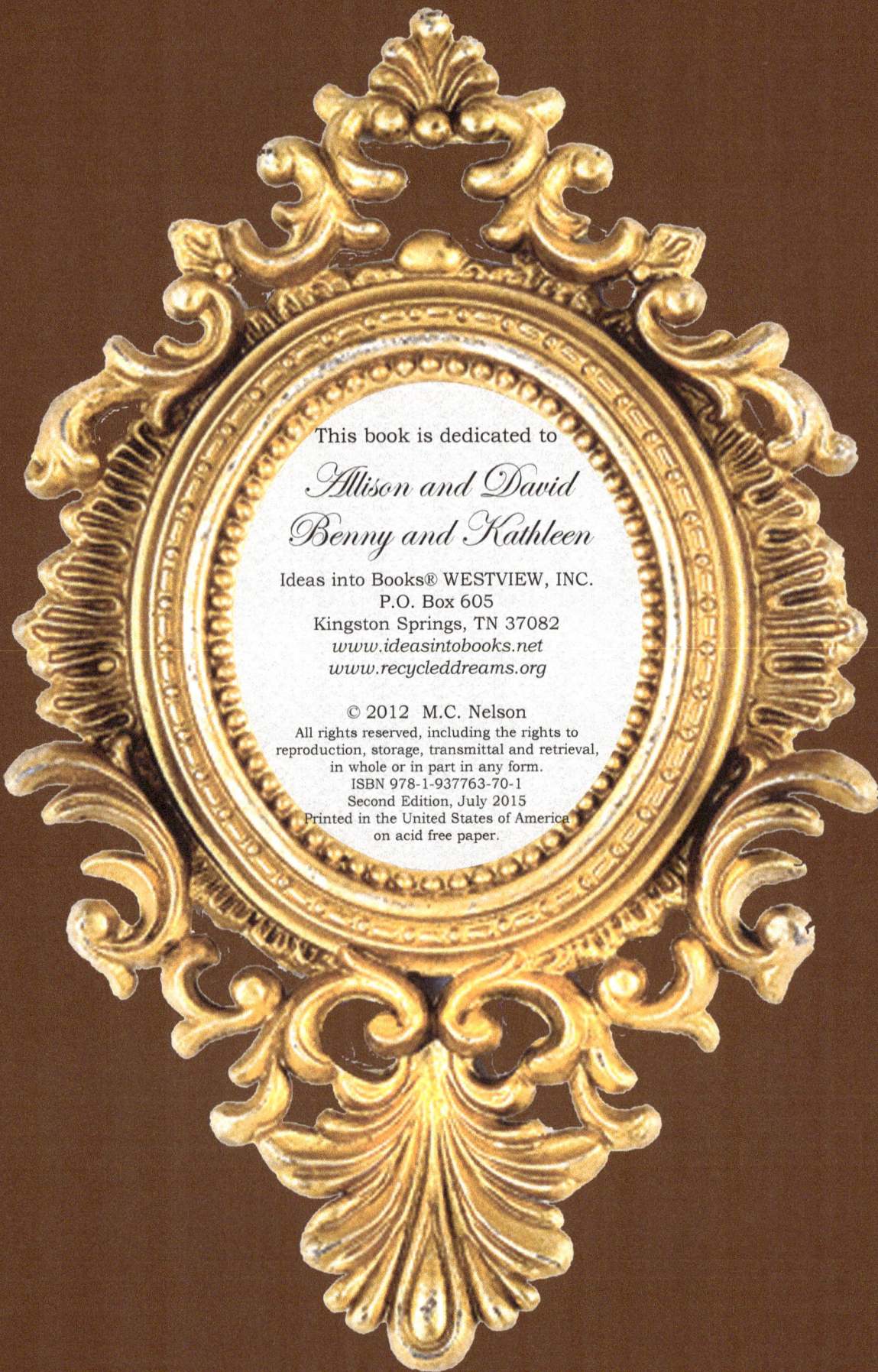

This book is dedicated to

*Allison and David*
*Benny and Kathleen*

Ideas into Books® WESTVIEW, INC.
P.O. Box 605
Kingston Springs, TN 37082
*www.ideasintobooks.net*
*www.recycleddreams.org*

© 2012  M.C. Nelson
All rights reserved, including the rights to
reproduction, storage, transmittal and retrieval,
in whole or in part in any form.
ISBN 978-1-937763-70-1
Second Edition, July 2015
Printed in the United States of America
on acid free paper.

The name given to me at birth:

I got that name because:

The date and place of my birth were:

My birth parents' names were:

My nicknames included:

I got those nicknames because:

I prefer to be called:

I was raised by:

My earliest memory is:

My mother's name at birth:

Place and date of my mother's birth:

My name for my mother:

My mother's name for me:

I would describe my mother as:

My mother's siblings were:

What I know about my mother's childhood:

What I know about my mother's adult life:

My father's name at birth:

Place and date of my father's birth:

My name for my father:

My father's name for me:

I would describe my father as:

My father's siblings were:

What I know about my father's childhood:

What I know about my father's adult life:

I remember about my mother:

My favorite thing about my mother:

Things my mother and I liked to do together:

My mother helped me feel most secure when:

The most important lesson I learned from my mother, and how I learned it:

Where, when, and how my mother died:

I remember about my father:

My favorite thing about my father:

Things my father and I liked to do together:

My father helped me feel the safest when:

The most important lesson I learned from my father, and how I learned it:

Where, when, and how my father died:

My mother's parents (my grandparents) were named:


I called that grandmother:

I called that grandfather:

My mother's parents called me:

They were originally from:


What I know about their lives:


My strongest memory of these grandparents:


The most important lesson I learned from these grandparents:


They died:

My father's parents (my grandparents) were named:


I called that grandmother:

I called that grandfather:

My father's parents called me:

They were originally from:


What I know about their lives:




My strongest memory of these grandparents:




The most important lesson I learned from these grandparents:




They died:

My mother's mother's parents (my great-grandparents) were named:

They came from:

As adults they lived:

What else I know about these great-grandparents:

My mother's father's parents (my great-grandparents) were named:

They came from:

As adults they lived:

What else I know about these great-grandparents:

My father's mother's parents (my great-grandparents) were named:

They came from:

As adults they lived:

What else I know about these great-grandparents:

My father's father's parents (my great-grandparents) were named:

They came from:

As adults they lived:

What else I know about these great-grandparents:

The names of my siblings and their birthdates:

I would describe my siblings this way:

When we were growing up, for fun we:

What our relationships are like now:

What I remember most about each of my siblings:

What I miss now about growing up with them:

What I know about the families they have now:

What I missed the most during my childhood:

The neighborhood I grew up in was:

I would describe it as:

Looks and smells and sounds I remember:

My best friends were:

Where my best friends lived:

What we liked to do together:

Other people I remember from my neighborhood, and what stands out about them:

The city closest to where I grew up was:



It could be described as:



It looked and sounded and smelled like:



What I remember about going to town as a child:



What we did when we went to town:

My favorite childhood memory:

This is how I would describe the house in which I grew up:

The inside was:

The outside was:

Looks and smells and sounds I remember:

The floor plan of the house in which I grew up:

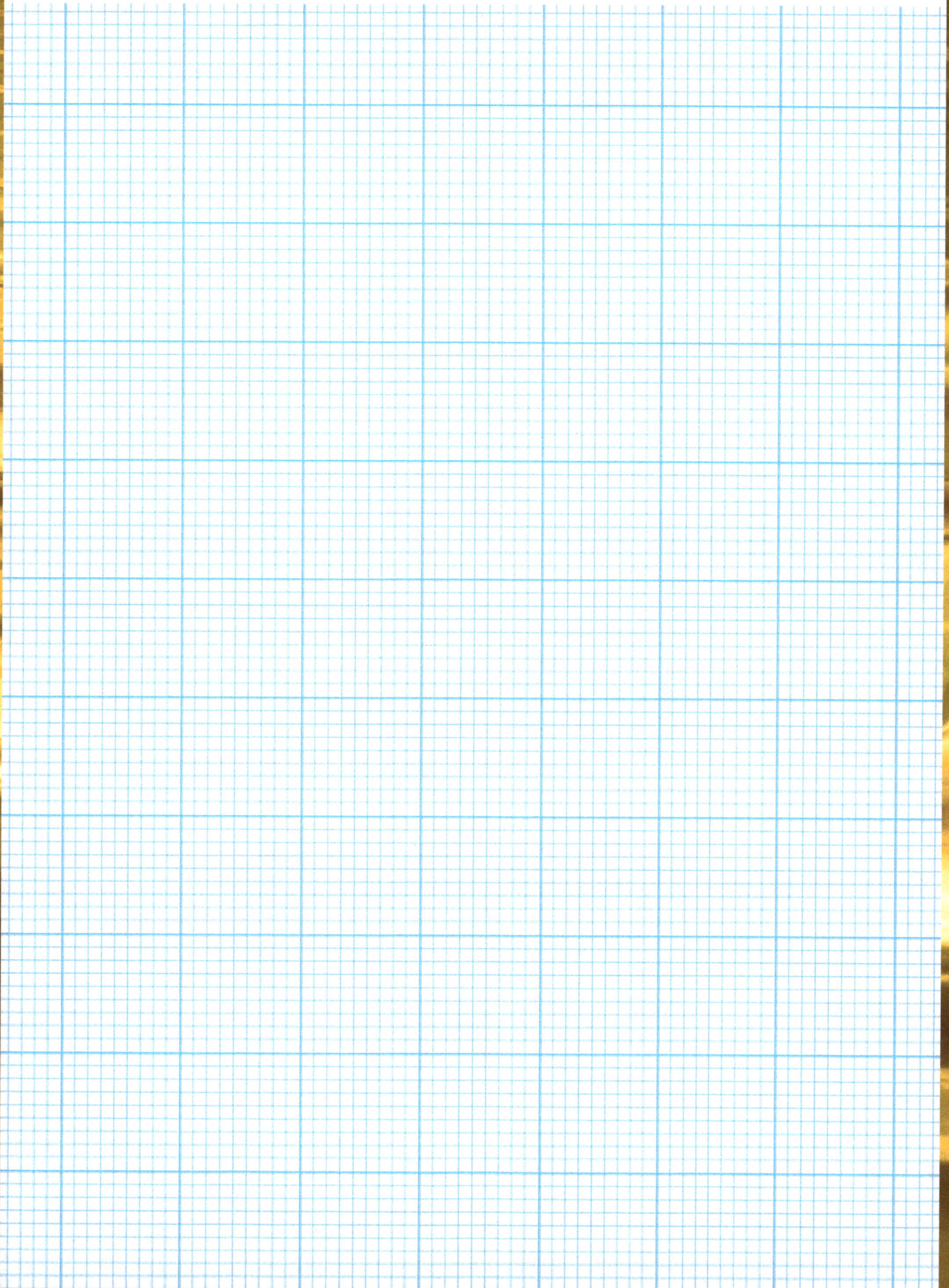

When I was a teenager, I lived:

My best friends were:

My responsibilities for work and chores were:

For fun, I:

I got into trouble when:

The best thing that happened to me was:

The worst thing that happened to me was:

When I was a teenager, these things were my favorites:

Music:
Musician:
Band:
Singer:
Actor:
Actress:
Movie:
Clothing:
Fashion:
Hero:
Subjects:
Food:

I was taught to drive by:

My first car was:

My worst accident was:

My first love was:

How we met:

What I remember about our courtship:

How it ended, if it did:

The greatest love of my life has been:

How we met:

What I remember about our courtship:

How it ended, if it did:

How I met my spouse:

My spouse's name:

Location of the wedding:

Who was there:

What the ceremony was like:

For our honeymoon, we went to:

(Give these details for each marriage.)

My spouse's occupation:

My spouse's favorite activity:

My in-law's names and where they came from:

What I know about my in-law's family:

That marriage lasted:

How it ended:

(Give these details for each marriage.)

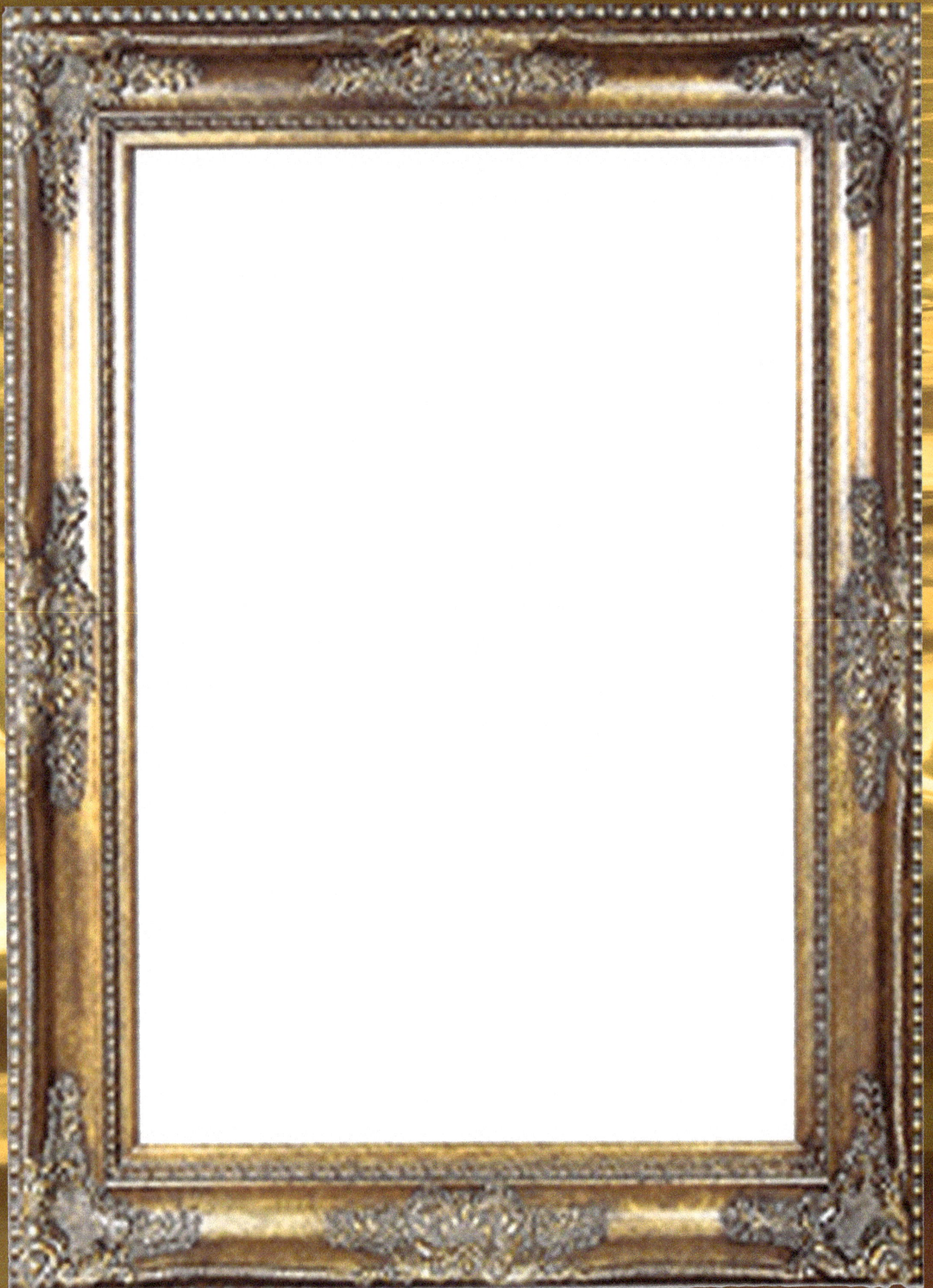

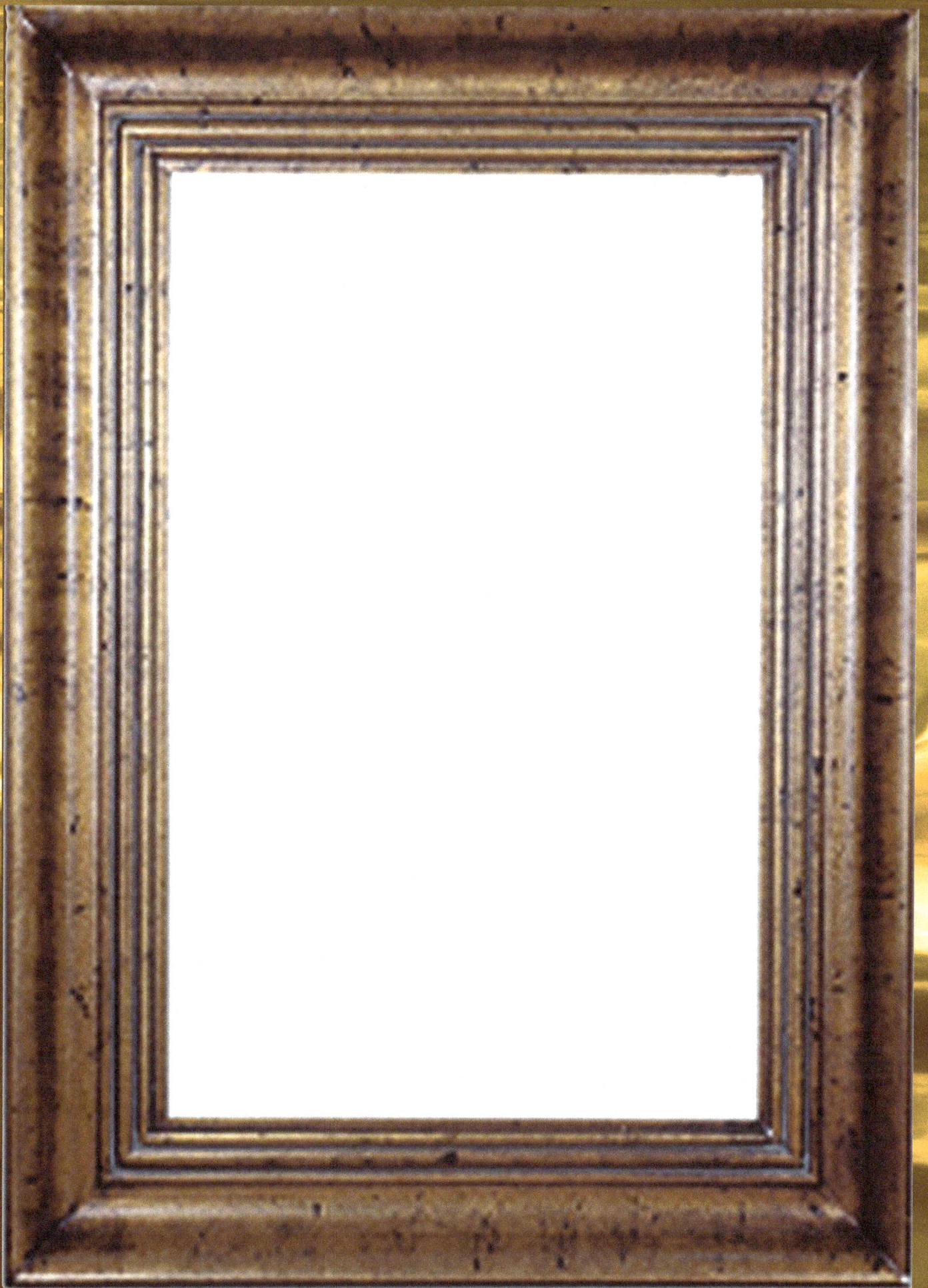

My children's names and birthdates:

My favorite memory of each one:

What our relationships are like today:

Where my children live now:

Activities my children are involved in now that they are adults:

Members of their families:

Let me tell you about my grandchildren:

Let me tell you about
my great-grandchildren:

My favorite way to celebrate my birthday when I was growing up:

My favorite way to celebrate my birthday now:

My favorite holiday and how I like to celebrate it:

My least favorite holiday, and why:

Hobbies I had growing up:

Hobbies I've enjoyed as an adult:

What I collect, and why:

How my collection started:

The animals that have been most important to me:




The pet I miss the most, and why:

What I remember about my elementary school:

What I remember about my teachers and my friends:

My most favorite elementary school activities:

My least favorite elementary school activities:

What I remember about my high school:

My best friends:

My easiest and most difficult subjects:

I celebrated my graduation by:

My first job after high school was:

Where I went for job training or post-high school education:


My major field of study:


My degree:


Where I went to graduate school:


There I studied:


Degrees and dates of graduation:


I paid for my education by:


My first job after I finished my education was:

Where and how my family worshiped when I was a child:

Who attended:

How often we went:

The part of the worship service that was the most meaningful to me then:

My deepest belief as a child was:

Why I believed as I did then:

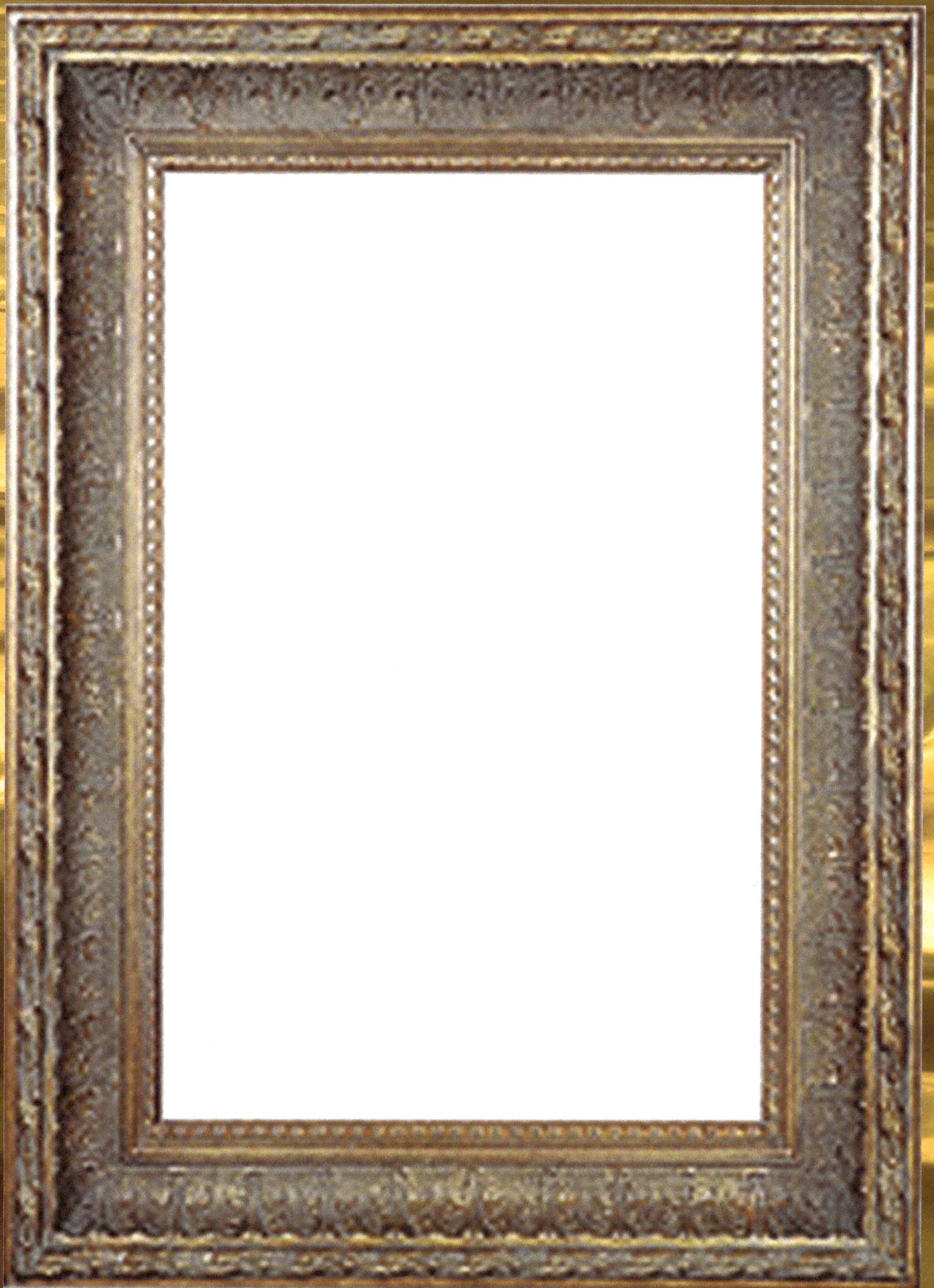

Where and how my family worships now:

Who attends:

How often we go:

The part of the worship service that is the most meaningful to me now:

My deepest belief now that I am an adult is:

Why I believe as I do now:

Military or volunteer service to my country:

Dates of service:

Branch of service:

Specialties:

Locations served:

My primary vocation has been:

My major responsibilities have included:

Responsibilities I most and least enjoyed:

My first home as an adult was:

My strongest memory of that place:

Most recently, I lived:

In my entire life, the place I lived the longest was:

What I remember about living there:

The floor plan of the house in which my children grew up:

The floor plan of my favorite house:

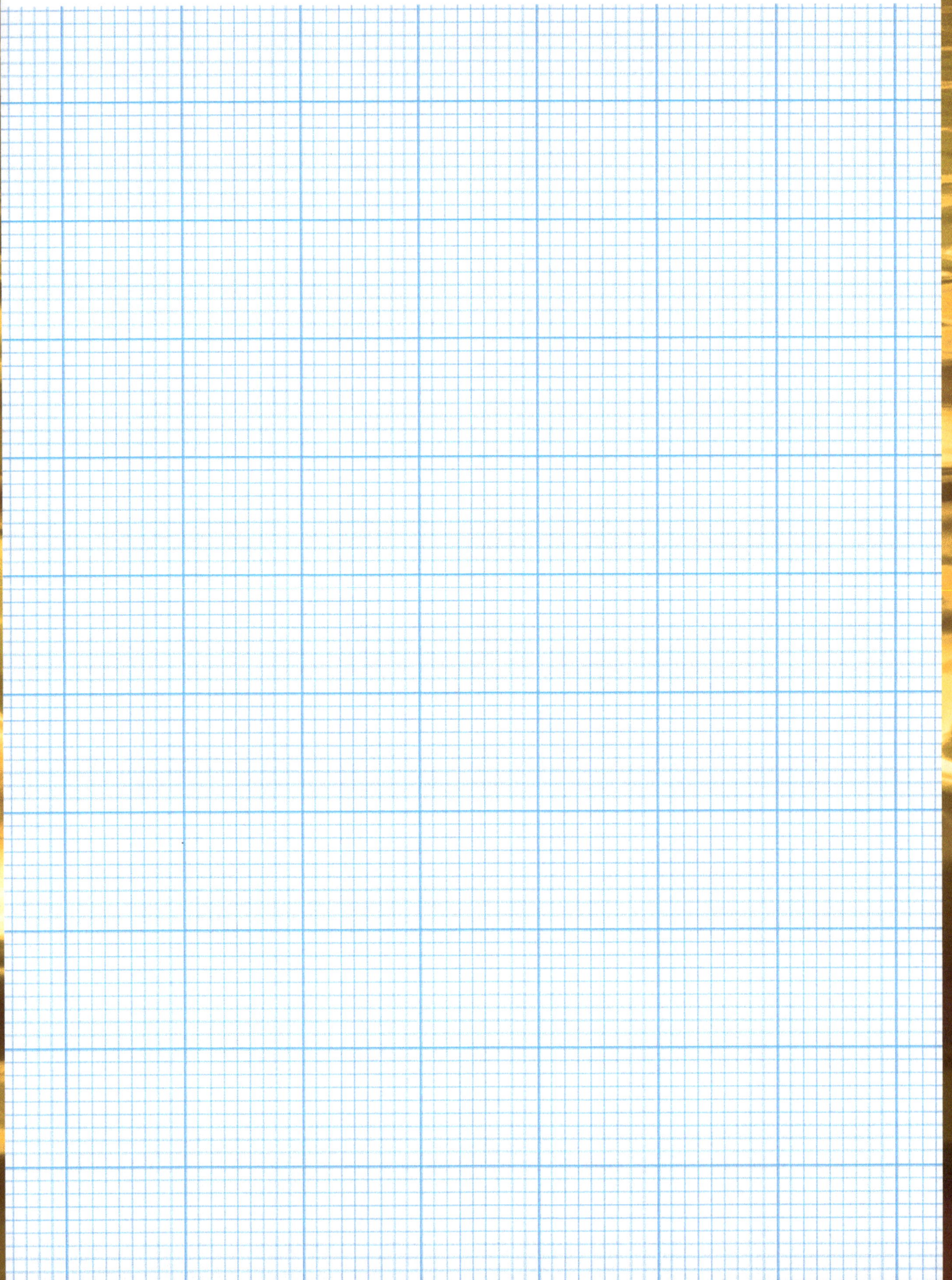

My favorite place I ever lived:

It was my favorite because:

It looked and smelled and sounded like:

I lived there with:

What I remember about living there:

Disabilities and adversities I've overcome include:

My special abilities include:

My favorite teacher was:

who taught me how to:

My favorite tradition:

My favorite daily routine:

My musical and artistic talents and gifts include:

My athletic talents and gifts include:

My academic talents and gifts include:

My creative talents and gifts include:

The event I am proudest of participating in:

Awards I've won include:

I learned to swim when:

Sports I played and the places I played them included:

Contests I won or placed in included:

I got my first bicycle when:

The farthest I ever rode was:

How it felt to be free:

The first car I paid for myself was:

I paid for it with money I earned by:

I had it until:

Other transportation I've owned or used includes:

My political beliefs include:

My civic and political activities have included:

I've been elected or appointed to the following offices:

I volunteered for these community activities:

I chose those activities because:

My responsibilities there included:

The happiest I've ever been in my life was when:

The best decision I ever made, and why it was:

The most miserable I ever was in my life and
how I got over it:

My biggest regret:

My favorite things:

Color:

Clothing:

Sport:

Team:

Weather:

Holiday:

Season:

Person:

Place:

Pastime:

Thing:

Soap:

Shampoo:

Deodorant:

Cologne:

Perfume:

Food:

Candy:

Condiment:

Beverage:

Dessert:

Snack:

Menu:

More favorite things:

Artist:

Artwork:

Author:

Book:

Instrument:

Musician:

Musical Composition:

Song:

Radio Show:

Television Star:

Television Show:

Movie Star:

Movie:

Hobby:

Toy:

Game:

Store:

Tree:

Flower:

Bird:

Animal:

Smell:

Sight:

Sound:

Building:

My closest friends throughout my life have been:

The things my friends and I
most enjoy doing together are:

My favorite vacation was going to:


when I was _____ years old.

The people who went with me were:



While I was there, we:



The very best part was:

Other places I have travelled and visited include:

My proudest moment was:

My most prized possession:

My three best memories have been:

The hardest thing I've ever lived through was:




What made it possible for me to survive was:

My favorite daily routine:

My favorite tradition:

My achievements have included:




I attribute my successes to:

Memorable things I've said or done include:

Funny things I've said or done include:

What I wish I had known at the time was:

It would have changed my life because:

What I would like others to know about me:




I would most like to be remembered for:

I learned the most valuable lesson of my life when:

Everything I've learned about things like getting along with other human beings, marriage, money, happiness, religion, raising kids, work, and love could all be summed up in these words:

The knowledge I'd most like to pass on is:

My best advice for future generations is:

The lives and historical events that had the most profound positive effect on me, and why, were:

The losses and traumatic events that had the most profound adverse effect on me, and why, were:

What makes me feel most valued is:

My greatest fears are:

The most frightened I have ever been was when:

What causes me the most stress is:

The thing that calms me down most easily is:

What I most like to do for fun is:

What I miss most is:

I am allergic to:

My worst allergic reaction was:

The sickest I have ever been was when:

The foods I dislike the most are:

What you can put on my food so I'll eat it:

The beverage I'm most likely to swallow my medication with is:

My favorite memory
of the owner of this book, written
by
_____.

My favorite memory
of the owner of this book, written
by
_____.

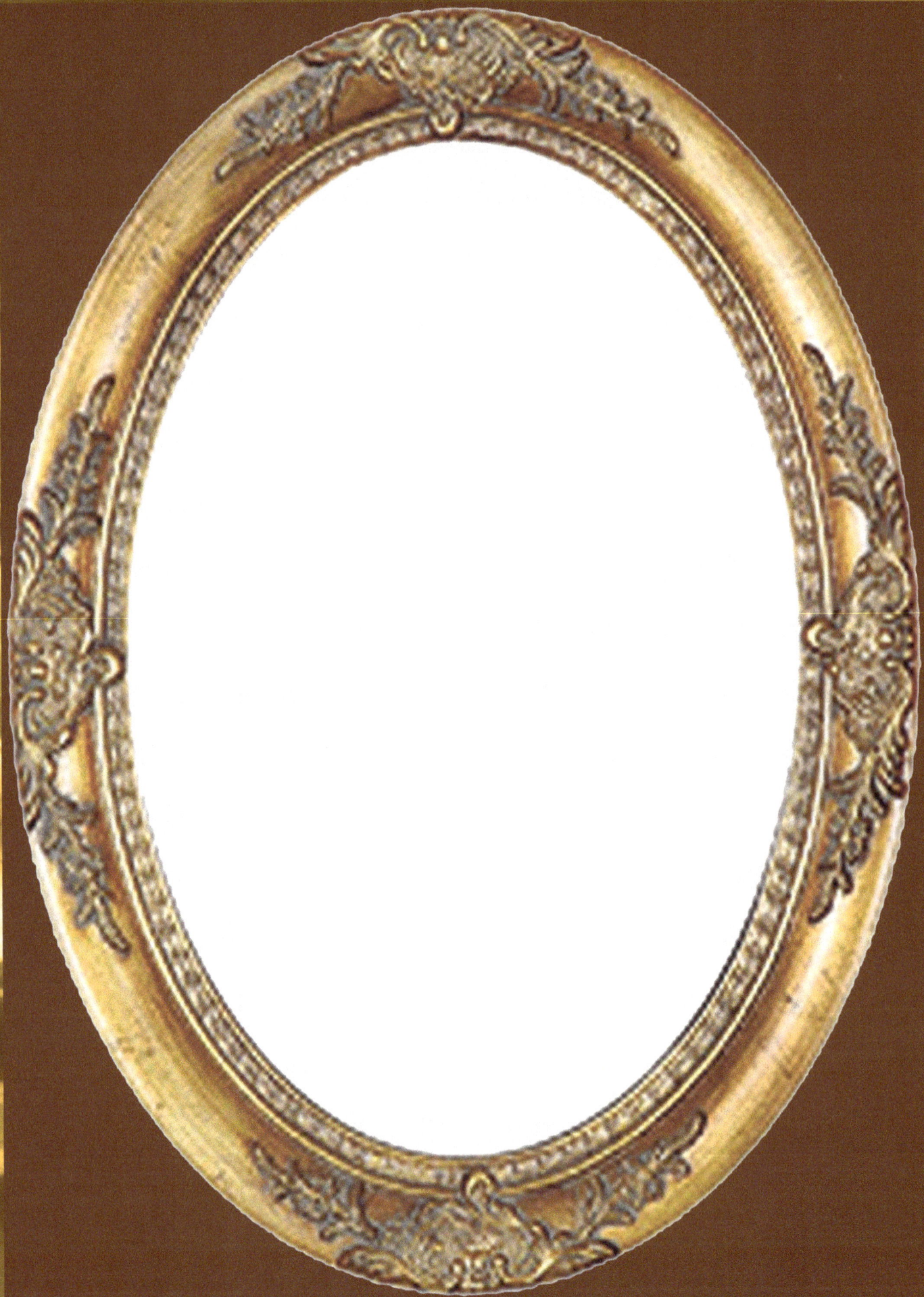

# Major Events Timeline

During my first twelve months:


When I was 1:


When I was 2:


When I was 3:


When I was 4:


When I was 5:


When I was 6:


When I was 7:


When I was 8:


When I was 9:


When I was 10:

# Major Events Timeline

When I was 11:

When I was 12:

When I was 13:

When I was 14:

When I was 15:

When I was 16:

When I was 17:

When I was 18:

When I was 19:

When I was 20:

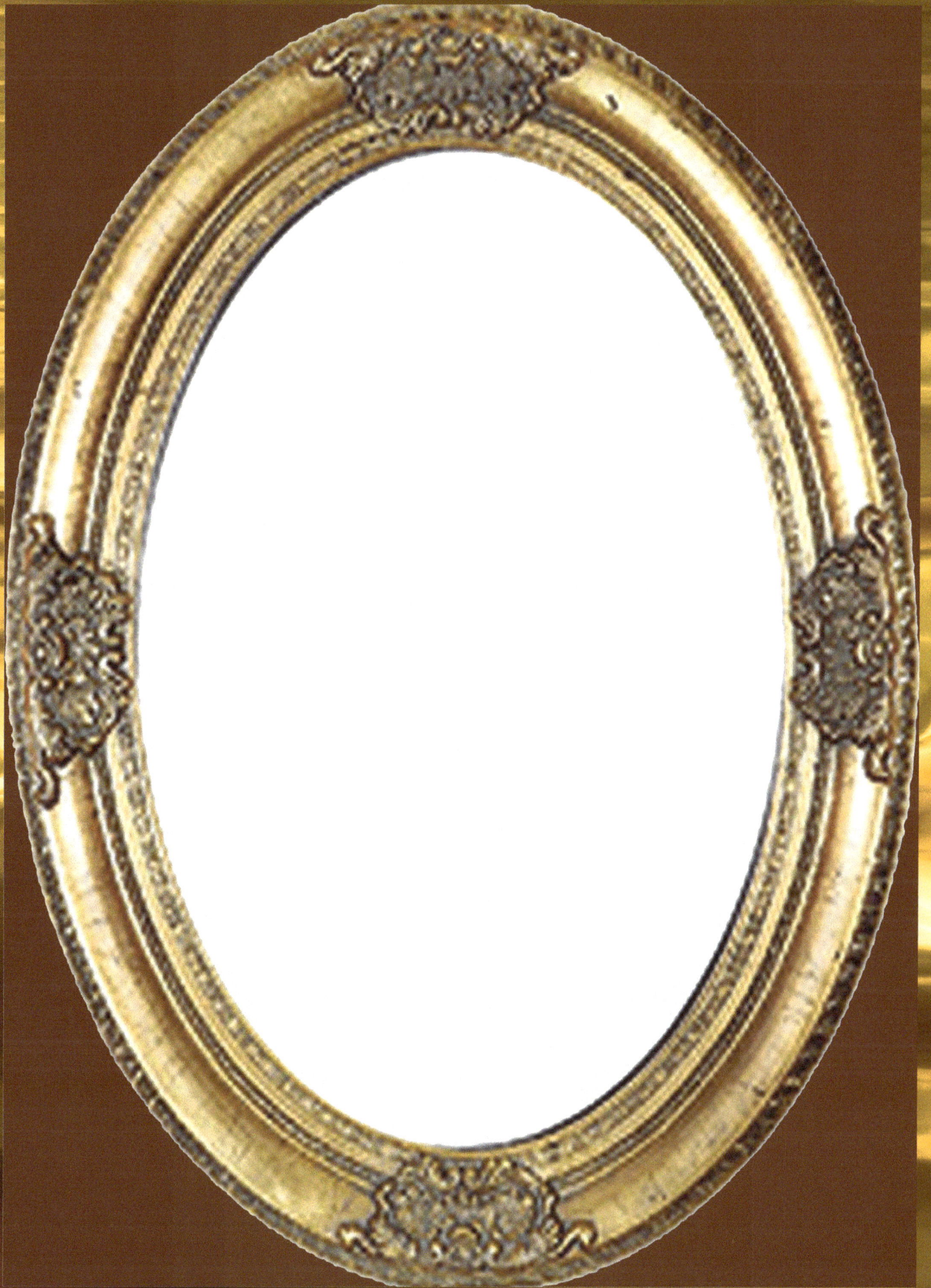

# Major Events Timeline

When I was 21:

When I was 22:

When I was 23:

When I was 24:

When I was 25:

When I was 26:

When I was 27:

When I was 28:

When I was 29:

When I was 30:

# Major Events Timeline

When I was 31:

When I was 32:

When I was 33:

When I was 34:

When I was 35:

When I was 36:

When I was 37:

When I was 38:

When I was 39:

When I was 40:

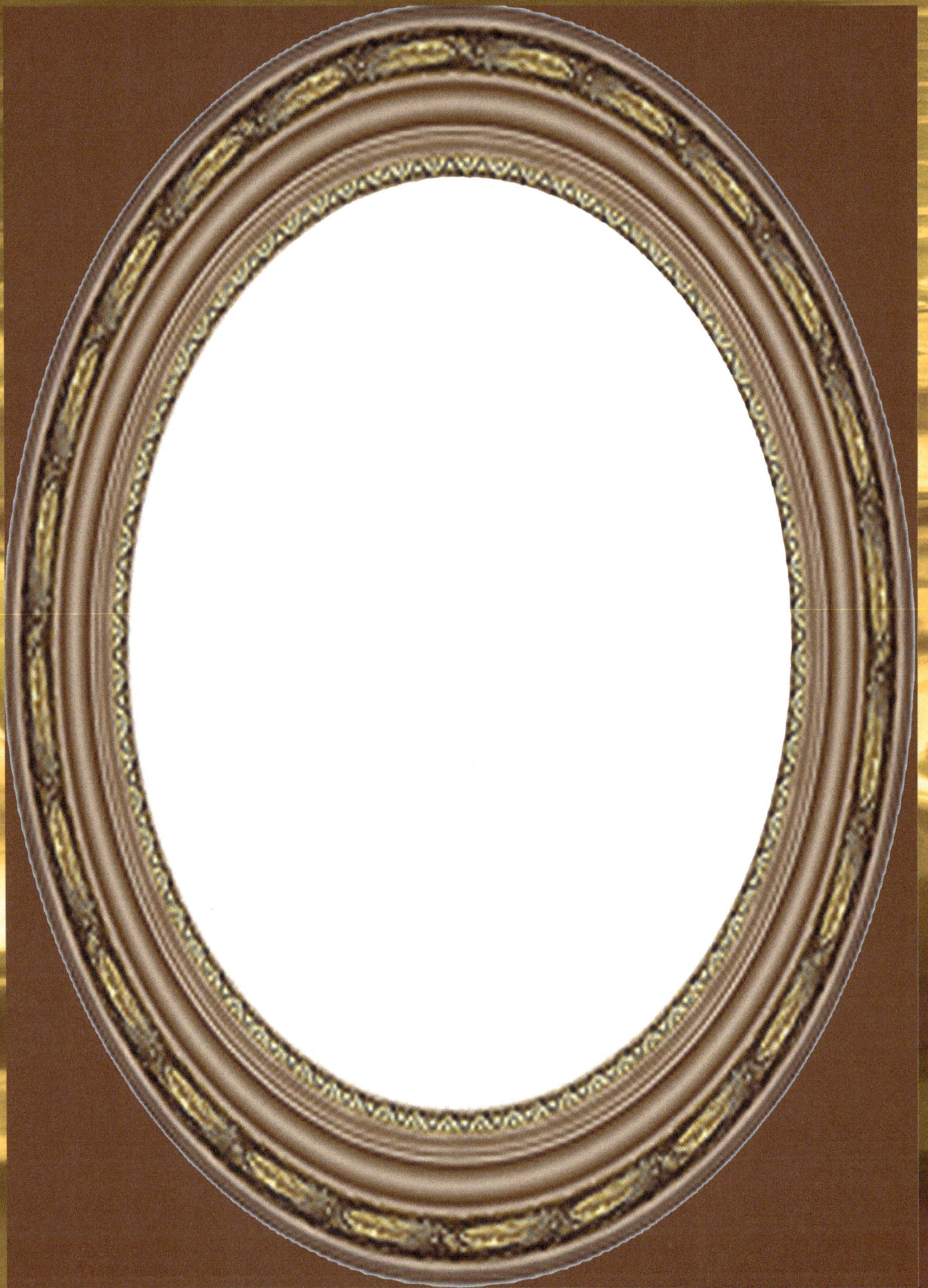

# Major Events Timeline

When I was 41:

When I was 42:

When I was 43:

When I was 44:

When I was 45:

When I was 46:

When I was 47:

When I was 48:

When I was 49:

When I was 50:

# Major Events Timeline

When I was 51:

When I was 52:

When I was 53:

When I was 54:

When I was 55:

When I was 56:

When I was 57:

When I was 58:

When I was 59:

When I was 60:

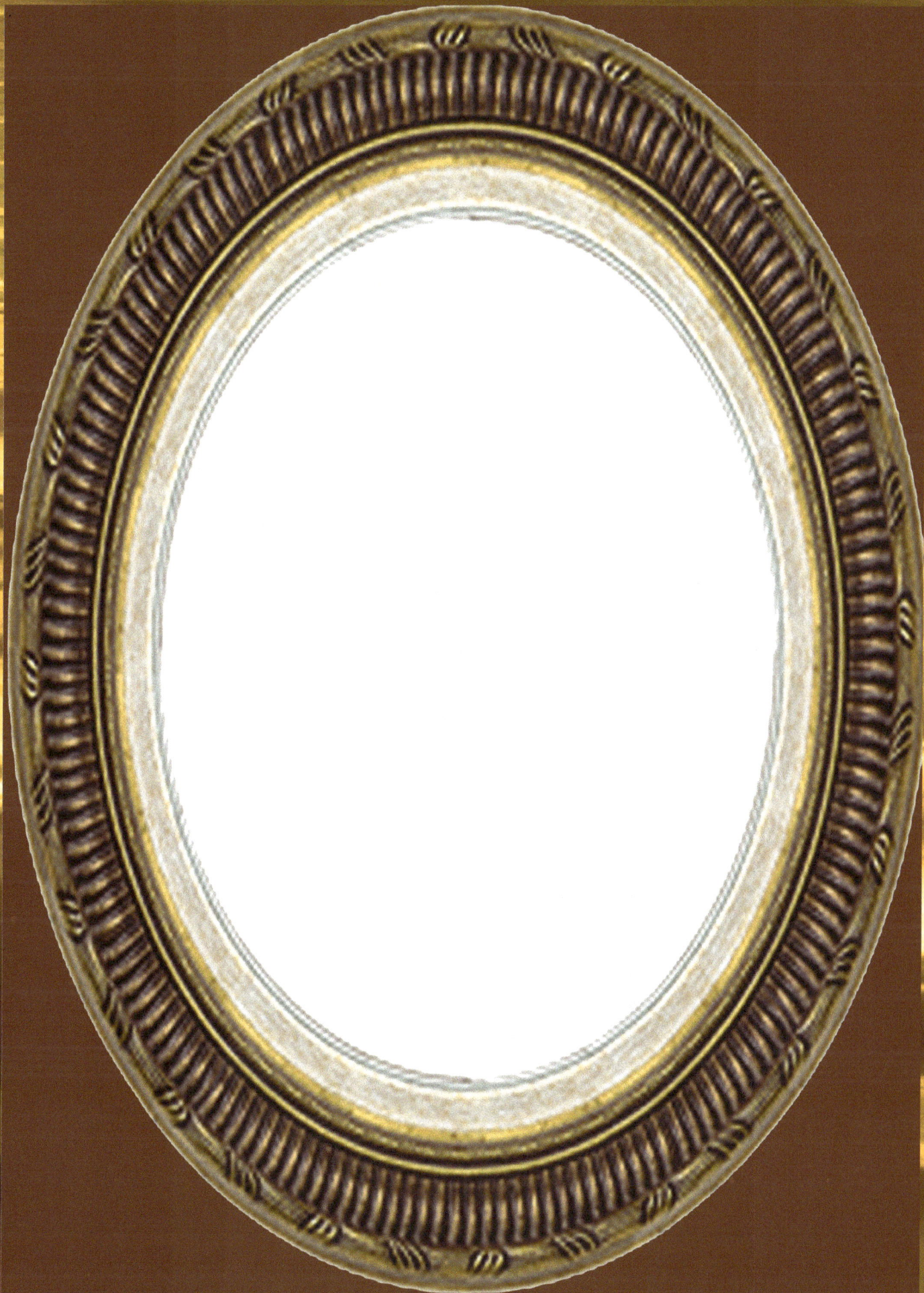

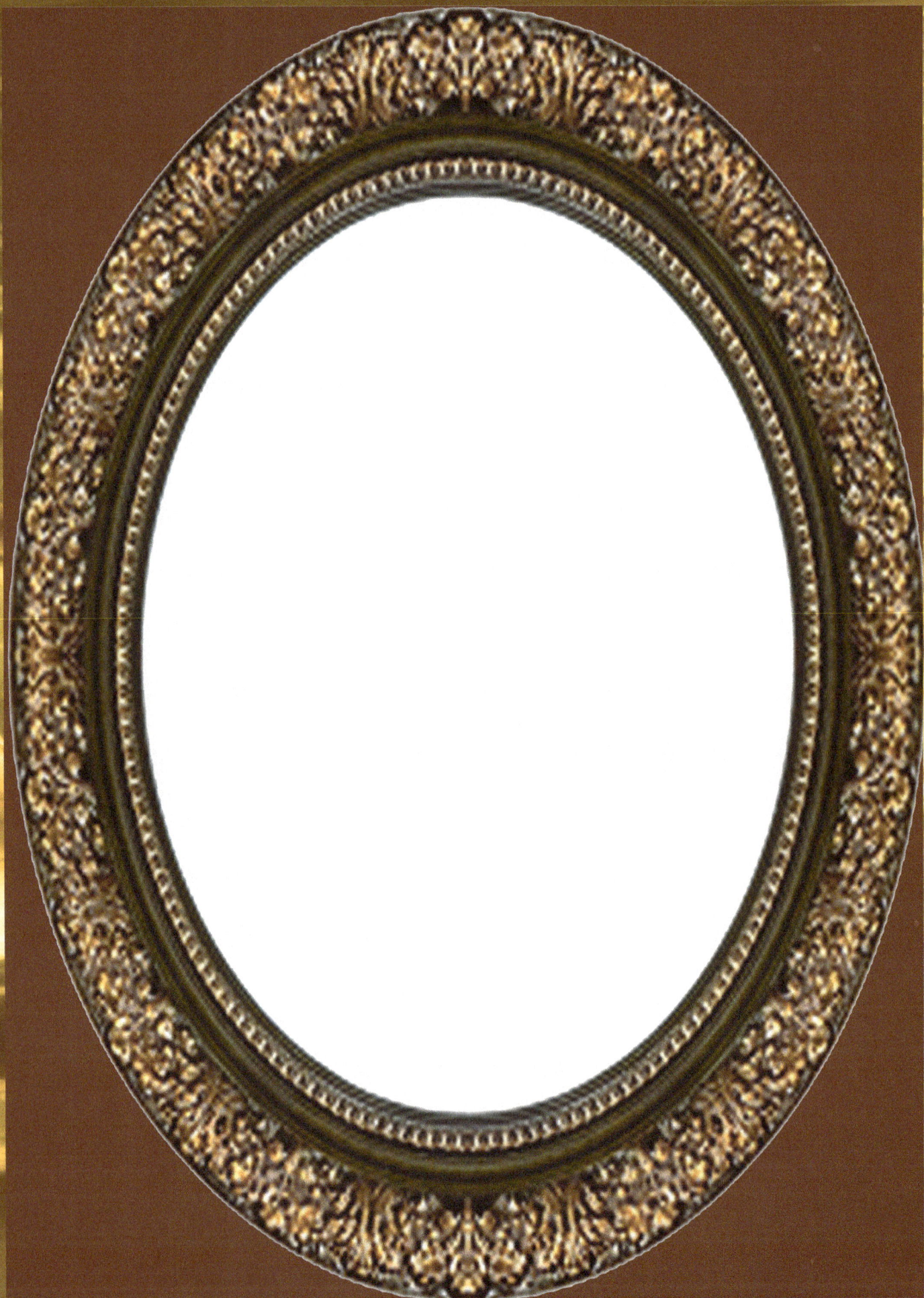

# Major Events Timeline

When I was 61:

When I was 62:

When I was 63:

When I was 64:

When I was 65:

When I was 66:

When I was 67:

When I was 68:

When I was 69:

When I was 70:

# Major Events Timeline

When I was 71:

When I was 72:

When I was 73:

When I was 74:

When I was 75:

When I was 76:

When I was 77:

When I was 78:

When I was 79:

When I was 80:

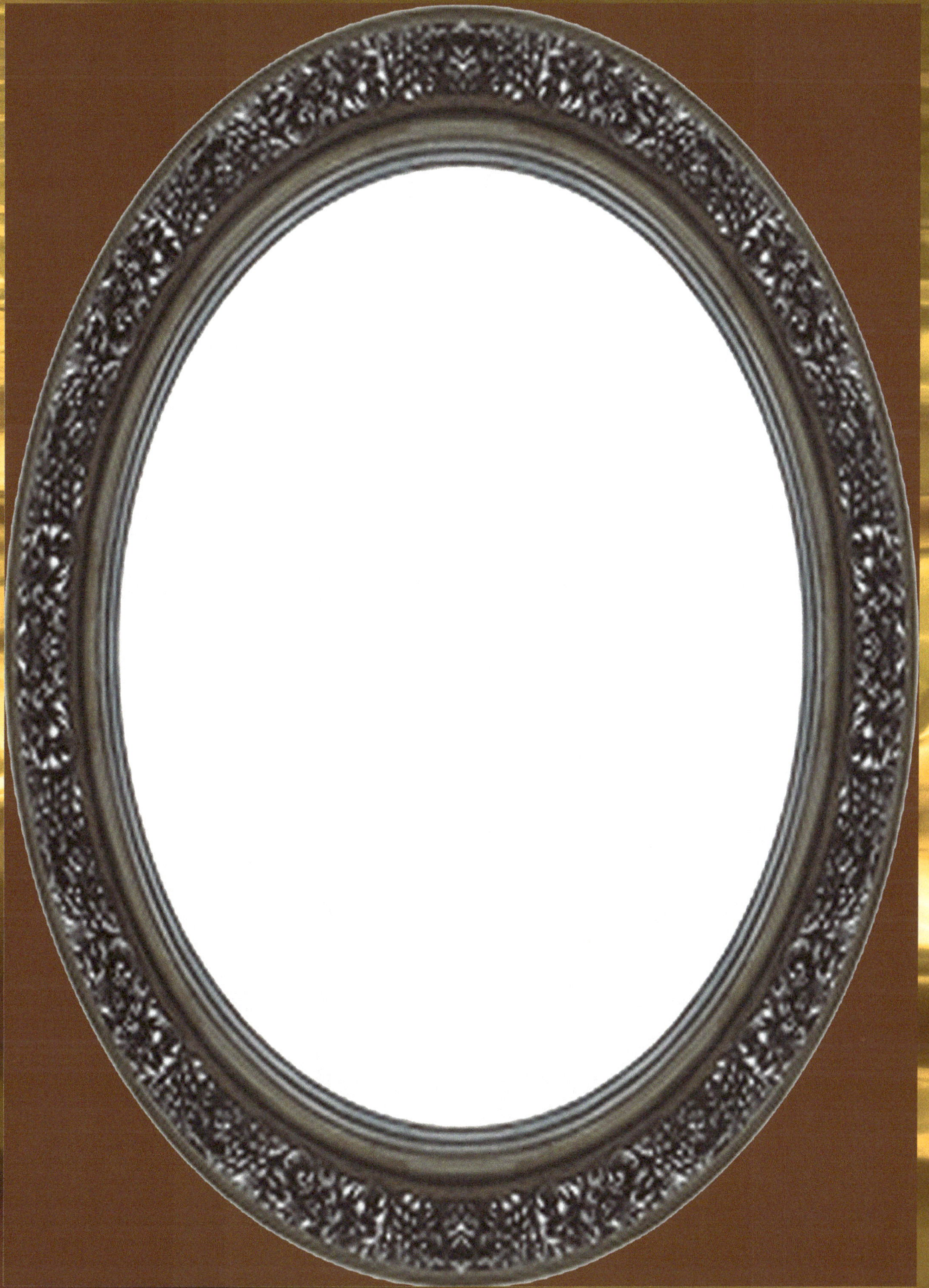

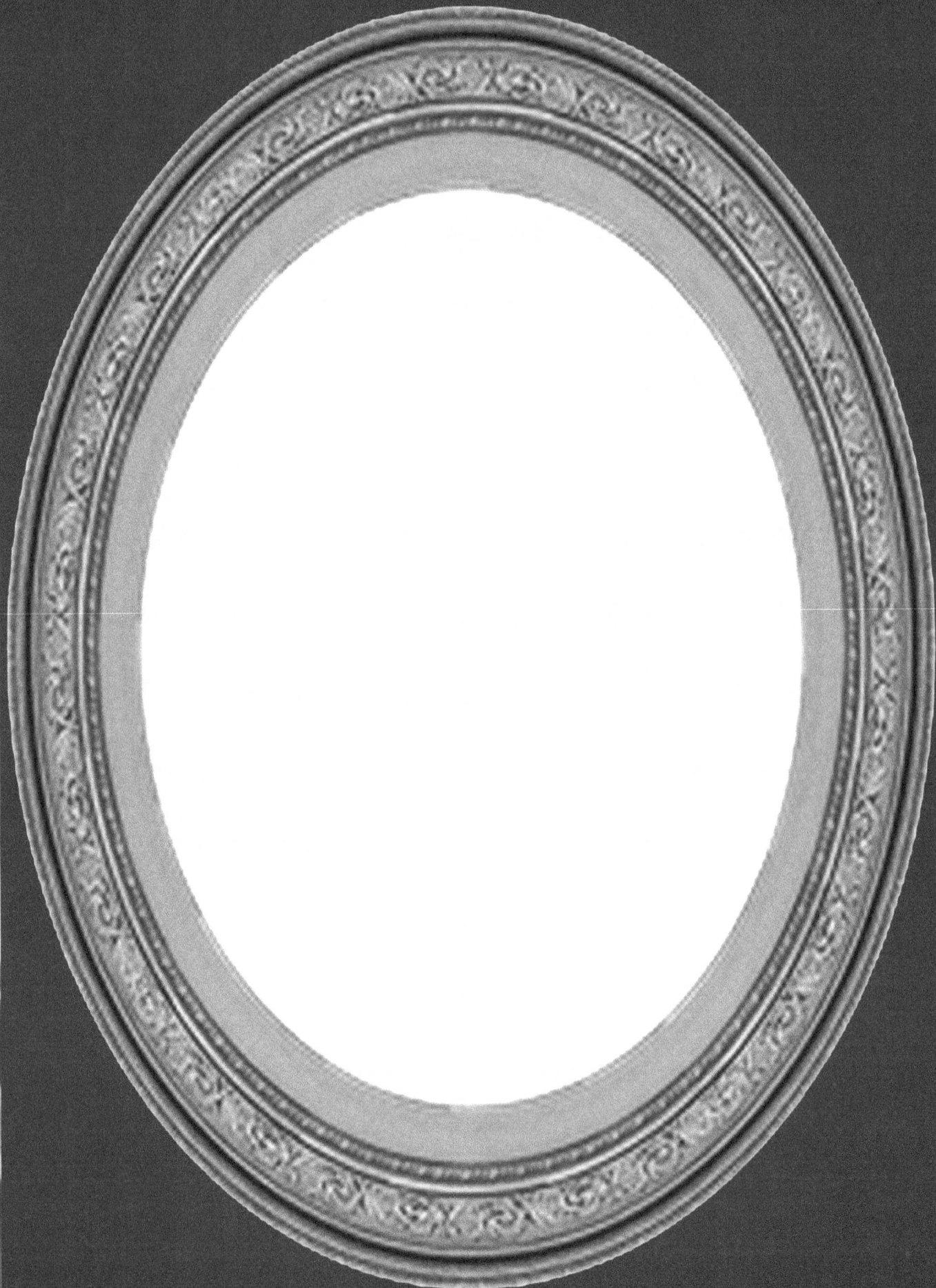

# Major Events Timeline

When I was 81:

When I was 82:

When I was 83:

When I was 84:

When I was 85:

When I was 86:

When I was 87:

When I was 88:

When I was 89:

When I was 90:

# Major Events Timeline

When I was 91:

When I was 92:

When I was 93:

When I was 94:

When I was 95:

When I was 96:

When I was 97:

When I was 98:

When I was 99:

When I was 100:

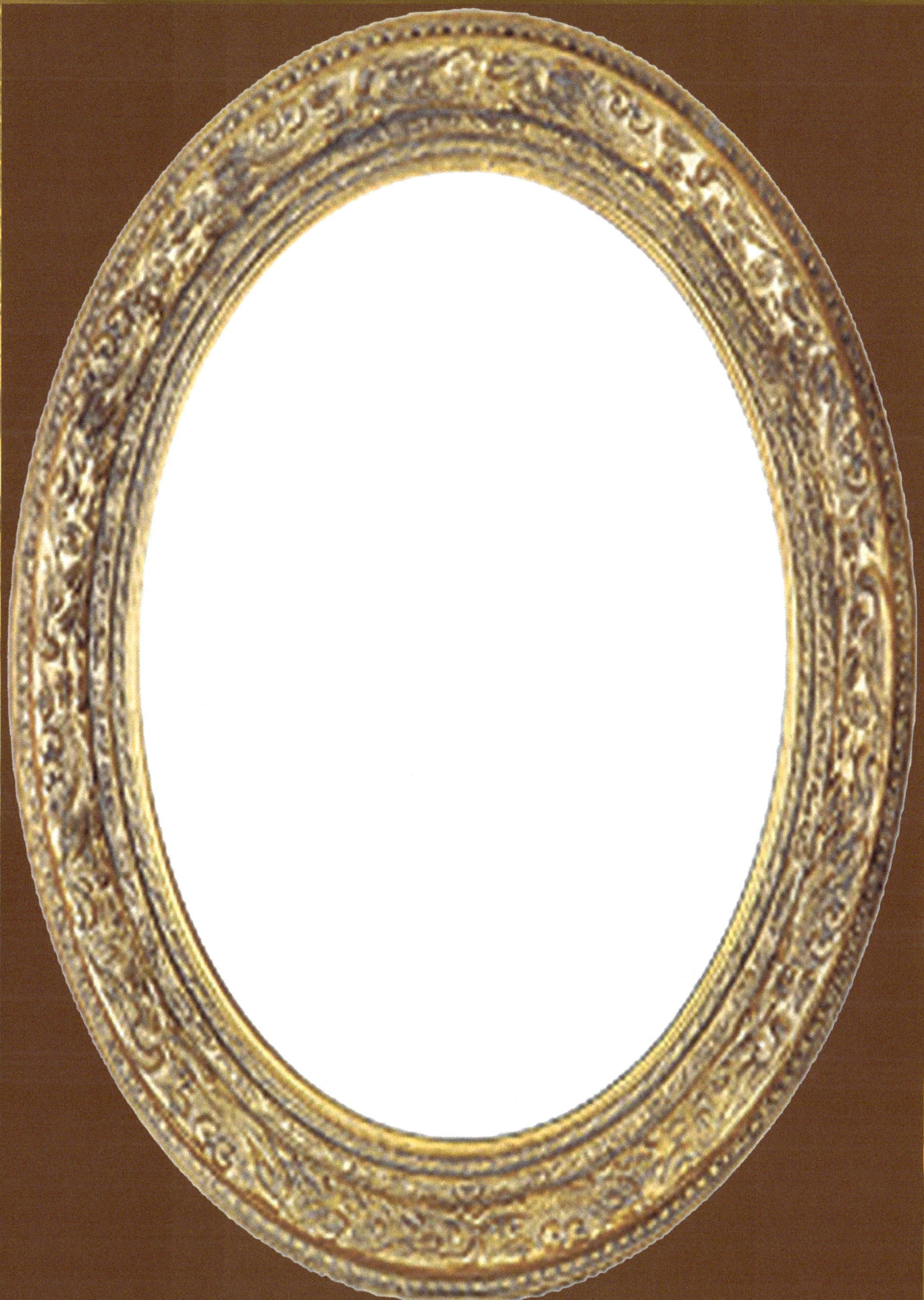

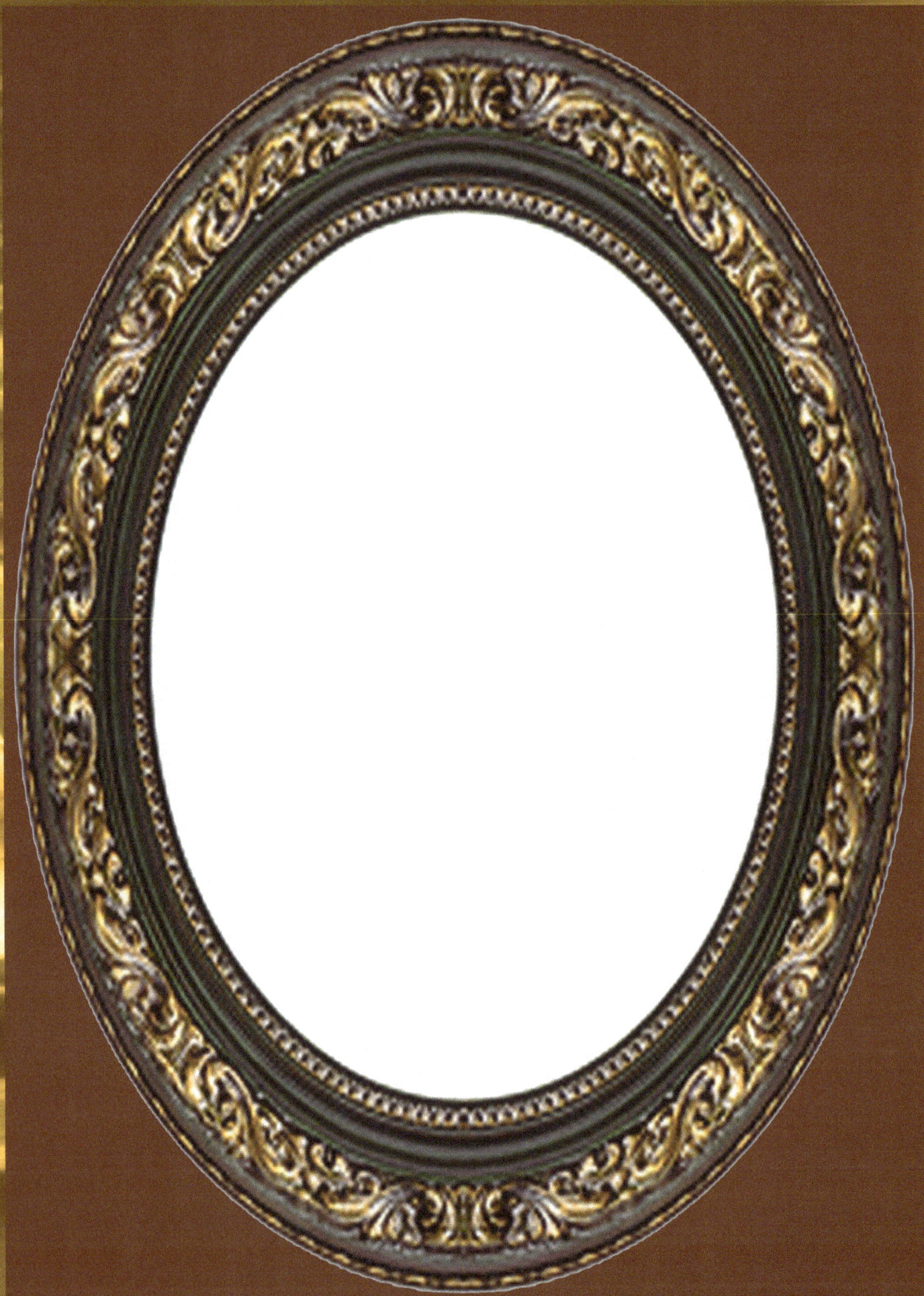

# Major Events Timeline

When I was 101:

When I was 102:

When I was 103:

When I was 104:

When I was 105:

When I was 106:

When I was 107:

When I was 108:

When I was 109:

When I was 110: